THINK 70/30:
HOW I LOST
100 POUNDS
AND KEPT IT OFF!

PLAIN AND SIMPLE
TECHNIQUES THAT
GET RESULTS

Shaun R

JONES MEDIA
PUBLISHING

TABLE OF CONTENTS

INTRODUCTION

I would like to share my life-changing journey of losing 100 pounds and keeping them off for over ten years. Most of the provided advice is diet and fitness-related information and knowledge I have learned over the years. When it comes to diet and fitness there is a lot of information available, but in chunks or concentrated on one topic. The idea is not to provide expanded information in lengthy story format, but instead remain concise while sharing the necessary key knowledge.

Good health is important. Without it life may not be so fun and enjoyable. In life, good health should be a priority and one should make it so for well-being.

Toward the end of most chapters there will be a brief summary of the highlights so they can be referred to again easily whenever needed. Weight loss will mainly refer to fat loss. Toward the end of the book there will be a table for keeping track of weight loss. Let's get started!

NUTRITION ESSENTIALS

Nutrition/diet is one of the most important factors when it comes to weight loss and a healthy lifestyle. Let's get started with the basics of nutrition. It's imperative to understand caloric breakdown and what food is generally comprised of: proteins, carbohydrates, and fats. See the following table for caloric breakdown.

	Proteins (1 gram)	Carbohydrates (1 gram)	Fats (1 gram)	Alcohol (1 gram)	Water (1 gram)
Calories	4	4	9	7	0

Take a moment to read this table one more time. Quick observation: one gram of fat contains a little over twice the number of calories when compared to one gram of protein and carbohydrate. Water is also listed in the table above, just as a reminder that it contains zero calories. We will expand on this later in the book.

Food products generally have a *Nutrition Facts* or *Information* label containing essential information. Depending on the type of food product, this label is typically located on the back of the packaging. Also, an *Ingredients List* is included. The significant aspect to know about the *Ingredients List* is the ingredients are listed in descending order from most to least (by weight). Meaning, the ingredient with largest weight or amount is listed first, and so on. Let's take yogurt as an example. If the second or third ingredient listed is sugar (or similar), then you know overall it is the second or third most prominent ingredient within the yogurt. Read through the entire list of ingredients to know and understand what exactly you may be consuming.

Now, before reading the calories, check the serving size to understand the quantity of that serving listed, shown by the *Servings Per Container* number. Calories listed are based on single (one) serving. Meaning, if there are 100 calories and three servings per container, and the entire food item is consumed (all three servings), then that would equate to a total of 300 calories (not 100). To calculate total calories, just multiply number of servings by calories listed. The nutrient content information is based on the serving size listed, so keep that in mind while reading the nutritional information.

The *Percent (%) Daily Value* on the *Nutrition Facts* label is typically based on a set amount of calorie diet—for example, 2,000 calories. Check the footnote toward the lower part of the *Nutrition Facts* label for specific information. This value is not for a single snack or meal, but instead one full day. In a day, one may consume less or more than 2,000 calories. Regardless, daily value percentage can be used as a guide or a frame of reference. Nutrient percentages over 20% should be considered thoughtfully based on overall diet.

To make an informed decision, I normally start with the ingredients list and take note of the first ingredient. Just as an example, when looking for a food product, if the first ingredient is listed as sugar, then I would not consume it, as sugar would be existing in the largest quantity (overall)—or if there is any other item on the ingredients list I would not like or not understand (like artificial preservatives), then the decision becomes easy before even reading the nutritional information. Otherwise, move on to reading the *Nutrition Facts* label.

On the *Nutrition Facts* label, the first thing I look at is the serving size and try to imagine the amount of the serving listed. For instance, whether it's one tablespoon (tbsp) or half a cup, by imagining, I roughly get an idea of how much it would be in quantity. Next, I look to see whether there are any trans fats, and if so, I would skip the food. Then I would note the amount of sodium and (added) sugar. Depending on how much I plan to consume in one go, while also keeping serving size in mind if either seems high to me—sodium around 20% daily value and/or sugar around 12g, which is about three teaspoons (tsp), I would most likely not go for it. Next, I check to see how much cholesterol there is (if any), specifically the percentage—if around 20% or higher I would think about it twice (depending on the type of food product it is and keeping the serving size in mind). Depending on overall diet plan and goals, view the remaining items such as total fat, carbohydrate, and protein to make a sound decision.

Glycemic index (GI) is basically a numerical value associated with foods on either how rapidly or slowly foods affect blood sugar (glucose) levels. The scale goes from 0 to 100 and is mainly for foods containing carbohydrates. Foods which have higher value on the scale (typically 70 or more) tend to release sugar (glucose) more quickly. Hence, these foods would tend to digest and absorb more rapidly. Consequently, foods with a lower value (typically 55 or less) on the scale tend to release sugar (glucose) gradually and can give a fuller feeling.

Food measurement. It is beneficial to know and understand food weights, quantities, and their correlation to understand the overall amount of food being consumed. One pound (456.59 gram) of most food items is approximately equal to two cups, or 16oz (ounces). Similarly, one tablespoon equals three teaspoons, and one cup equals 16 tablespoons.

Let's take a couple examples. When buying one pound of ground beef, it's a quick and easy conversion to approximately two cups, which can yield four quarter-pound burger patties. Furthermore, doing a quick internet search for calorie and nutrition breakdown can provide even more information per serving. Secondly, one tablespoon of granulated sugar converts to approximately 12.5g (gram). As an example, when buying a candy bar, if the nutrition label mentions 25g of sugar, then doing a quick conversion from grams to tablespoons would mean it contains two tablespoons of sugar.

✦ **TIP:** It can be very helpful to at least observe measuring cups, tablespoons, and teaspoons (or similar) in person or buy them for at-home cooking. The idea is to be able to correlate weight to quantity or amount when buying or consuming food and have an overall idea of conversions and measurements. For example, looking at one or more tablespoons of sugar in person and seeing how much in quantity it actually is to obtain a perspective.

As listed on the caloric breakdown table, one gram of alcohol has approximately seven calories, and has no nutritional value. The assumption is our body cannot store alcohol, therefore has to burn it or get rid of it, resulting in disruption of other processes such as fat burning and perhaps nutrient absorption. Many health and fitness experts do not drink or smoke and stay healthy.

Brief Summary:

- Refer to the following table for understanding caloric breakdown.

	Proteins (1 gram)	Carbohydrates (1 gram)	Fats (1 gram)	Alcohol (1 gram)	Water (1 gram)
Calories	4	4	9	7	0

- Read and understand the *Nutrition Facts* label, referring to the associated percentages as a general guideline and remembering it's per serving (or as specified).
- Carefully read the ingredients list.
  - Ingredients are listed in descending order (by weight) from most to least.
- Know glycemic index and glycemic load in relation to food.
- Food measurements can be important and helpful.

JOURNEY TOWARD LOSING 100 POUNDS

G rowing up, I was an overweight kid. Life was quite different back then with those extra pounds being carried around. In those days, I never recognized nor realized I was overweight. Thinking back, during my early teens, however, I was able to perform physical activities without getting tired. It seemed to not impact or affect any of my routine during my younger life. I never weighed myself when younger, so was unsure of my weight at that time.

Back then, people would randomly share tips and suggestions on how to lose weight. I would try for few days, then would casually go back to my normal routine. When I started to think about it with a little more seriousness, I created a chart with a schedule to run every morning, and based on a suggestion, drink one to two glasses of water before a meal. I tried this plan for about a week without consistency or seriousness and went back to my normal routine. Afterward, I started going to the gym and still was not able to achieve any results.

Not until my late teens did I realize I was overweight. Consequently, one day I just literally got tired of the way I felt, how much food I ate every day, and how I looked, while also thinking about potential health-related concerns due to being overweight. That very same day I started with seriousness. I was twenty years old. I sort of had an idea my extra weight was mainly due to the type and amount of food I ate. Also, I had previously done a little bit of internet research on weight (fat) loss, but never had really given those diets a try. Therefore, the day I started the first thing I did was change the type of food I was eating. I weighed myself and took note and used a calendar to keep track of my weight, and began going to the gym twice a day, early in the morning and evening. Thinking back now, making the change in diet mainly helped—it was generally low carbohydrates, and overall calories were lower than maintenance calories. And I remember when I started, I did not count overall calories consumed in a day.

It was challenging in the beginning, as it was a sudden and significant change of diet for me. I had to stay strong during the first few days, then it felt like I began to get used to the change. What further assisted was after the initial few days I weighed myself and had lost approximately four pounds. It was an exciting feeling and helped me even more with motivation. Keeping the initial results in mind while using strong focus and willpower, I said no to fast food, soda, and desserts (or foods with added sugar). I would weigh myself every three days or so and keep note on a paper calendar. Weight loss continued at a steady pace, approximately around two, sometimes up to three pounds a week for the first three months. Then it felt like I had reached a plateau. Frequency of weight loss became quite slow. That's when I learned I had to modify my diet and routine to establish a change from the consistent diet I got used to following. The weight loss became more gradual, approximately one to two pounds a week. I would barely eat out, choosing instead to cook and prepare meals at home.

There used to be random days when I would go off track with my diet and overeat (sort of like a cheat meal)—for example, have desserts and eat fast food. It would result in a weight gain of approximately one to three pounds. On the following day, I would then sometimes have a slight urge to overeat again, however, would maintain strong focus and got back on track with the diet. The one to three pounds of weight gain would, on average, take a week or less to lose.

During my weight loss journey, I was in college. Sometimes I would go to the gym on campus, and one day found out they offered a personal training course. It caught my interest, and during the summer I took the full personal training course. It was a great learning experience. I also had discussions with doctors about losing weight and diet, and spoke with friends and family who had tried or were into a healthy diet and fitness.

Ten years later, I still remember how much I weighed back when I started: 297 pounds. Over a period of approximately a year and a half I lost a little over 100 pounds and got down to 194 pounds (height 5'11"). That is when I felt I had accomplished something. I simply felt great, and the results were just amazing. I have managed to keep the excess weight off for ten years, with my weight now hovering around 180 pounds.

DIET

Prior to losing weight, my diet was mainly comprised of fast, processed foods, sodas, and desserts. When I started losing weight, and based on the limited information I had related to weight-loss diets, I started with eating lean proteins such as canned tuna, grilled and/ or boiled chicken, and fish. I reduced fats and carbohydrates, and weight started to shed. After learning about glycemic index (GI), I mainly chose carbohydrates with low and medium GI (except for fruits and vegetables). About three months in, I also reduced sodium/salt intake.

Occasionally, the food I was eating felt bland without much flavor, especially vegetables, so I researched and created a supplementary food item list to bring a little flavor to the food and not get tired of similar tasting meal repetition. I had also printed a copy of this list and attached it on the refrigerator for reference. With time I enhanced this list, and it's included below.

My Diet Plan

I consumed a minimum of four, and up to six, meals a day. Timing of meals was usually two to three hours after a meal or certain time after when I felt hungry. Water intake of three to four liters (spread throughout the day), no alcohol or smoking, low (added) sugar and salt/sodium consumption.

Meal 1 – *Morning/Breakfast:*
Protein: 20-30g, Carbs: 20-30g, Fat: about 8-12g

Meal 2 – *Late Morning/Early Afternoon:*
Protein: 25-35g, Carbs: 20-30g, Fat: about 8-12g

Meal 3 – *Mid/Late Afternoon:*
Protein: 25-35g, Carbs: 15-20g, Fat: about 7-9g

Meal 4 – *Late Afternoon:*
Protein: 20-30g, Carbs: 15-20g, Fat: about 7-9g

Meal 5 – *Evening:*
Protein: 25-35g, Carbs: 10-15g, Fat: about 7-9g

Meal 6 – *Evening/Night:*
Protein: 15-25g, Carbs: 5-10g, Fat: about 1-2g

*Protein, carb, and fat values are approximate.

Carbs (Carbohydrates): Whole grains, brown rice, white rice, whole wheat (bread), oatmeal, whole oats, popcorn without butter/cheese and unsalted, beans, legumes. Sometimes green tea over coffee without sugar, milk, yogurt, Greek yogurt. Fruits such as apple, banana, orange, grapefruit, peach. Vegetables such as spinach, broccoli, cauliflower, carrots, mushrooms, Brussel sprouts, cabbage, cucumber.

Protein: Grilled, steamed, or boiled fish (preferably wild caught), canned salmon or tuna, eggs*, turkey, chicken*, lamb/goat (lean, low fat), beef (lean, low fat). *Organic*

Fat: Extra virgin olive oil, coconut oil, almonds, peanuts, cashews, other nuts, omega-3/fish oil, avocado.

My normal routine would be to wake up around 6:30 AM and head to a gym, where I would do intense cardio for about ten to fifteen minutes followed by about twenty to thirty minutes of resistance/weight training. After returning from the gym, have breakfast, shower, and leave for college/class. I would prepare my meals in advance and take them with me to minimize eating out. Two to four hours later, depending on the class schedule, have lunch, followed by a late afternoon meal or a snack a few hours later. I would carry a water bottle and drink plenty of water throughout the day (even when not thirsty). Depending on how I felt during the day, I would have a healthy snack in between meals as well. After returning home, I would eat dinner, timed at least two hours before bedtime. After first few months, as time allowed, I would go for about ten to fifteen minutes of continuous walk after dinner. I slept eight hours on average.

The key was to prepare meals in bulk and in advance. Most of the planning and meal preparation was done over the weekends, some being at night during weekdays as needed. Meals were stored in plastic or glass containers in the fridge in a ready-to-go state. For longer storage I would sometimes use the freezer.

There were times I would not lose weight at the time of weigh in. That was okay, as it came off eventually over the next few weeks. After about three months it felt I reached a plateau, and I tried to modify the diet. I would adjust, changing/reducing overall salt/sodium and carbohydrate intake, trying other types of food and recipes, changing exercise routine, adjust overall calories (eating a little less or a little more with some meals). I tried increasing my protein intake to one gram of protein per pound of body weight, which for me was a lot of protein. I was not very successful at it, mainly due to trying to eat high volumes of protein throughout the day, which was not enjoyable.

For a brief period I used to have a post-workout protein shake. It was a pure whey protein supplement (low carb). After focusing on the meaning of the word supplement, I thought, *Is that necessary?* With or without, I did not see any differences overall, and afterward realized it's also processed, so I did not continue using it.

Throughout, some of my knowledge was learning by trial and error, but the key was remaining focused and consistent. And weight would eventually continue to shed. I forced myself to have healthy food options for snacking, meals prepared and readily available so unhealthy snacks did not become an option. I simply just didn't buy the unhealthy foods. Back then I also did not know much about counting calories, I just kept a close watch on what I ate.

BRIEF SUMMARY:

- Diet is one of the key elements when it comes to weight loss.
- Be mindful about food choices.
- Utilize advanced food preparation.
- Be focused, disciplined, and patient.
- Dieting can be a very helpful learning experience.

Supplementary Food Item List

- Lemon
- Yellow mustard
- Vinegar
- Spices, herbs, and seasonings *(with low or no salt/sodium)*
  - Garlic, ginger, pepper, turmeric, cinnamon, basil, cilantro, oregano, parsley, mint, etc.
- Organic mayonnaise *(in small quantities, around ½ tablespoon or less)*
- Organic ketchup *(in moderate quantity, around ½ tablespoon)*
- Honey—raw, pure, or organic *(in moderate quantity, around ½ tablespoon or less)*
- Extra virgin olive oil *(in moderate quantity, ½ tablespoon or less)*
- Coconut oil *(in moderate quantity, ½ tablespoon or less)*
- Organic butter *(in moderate quantity, ½ tablespoon or less)*
- Organic almond or peanut butter *(in moderate quantity, ½ – one tablespoon)*
- Sea salt or Himalayan pink salt *(in very small quantities)*
- Salsa *(homemade preferred)*

SNACKS

- Organic granola or similar bars *(avoiding ones with high added sugar content or high fructose corn syrup)*
- Almonds, peanuts, cashews, or other nuts
- Plain Greek yogurt *(unflavored with added fruit or a little honey)*
- Organic cheese *(in small quantities)*
- Popcorn *(Non-GMO or organic, avoid microwave popcorn)*
- Sparkling or soda water, plain or add lemon/lime *(substitute for sodas)*
- Coconut water
- Fruit/vegetable smoothies *(in moderate quantity, without added sugar/ sweetener)*
- Fruit Juice *(100% pure, not from concentrate, in small quantities to avoid too much fruit sugar content)*
- Fruits *(apple, banana, orange, grapefruit, peach, avocado, dates, etc.)*
- Home-baked items such as banana bread, without sugar, substitute with honey in small quantity
- Whole potato or sweet potato chips *(kettle cooked or baked)* ones with relatively lower sodium and oil/fat *(in moderate quantity)*

✦ **Tip:** Always wash hands before eating, and also wash fruits and vegetables before eating.

✦ **Tip:** Do not forget to drink plenty of water throughout the day.

✦ **Tip:** Keep some of the snacks and other healthier items at home and take some snacks to go to have handy options.

TYPE OF DIETS TRIED

Aside from the multi-meal diet (five or more meals a day), there are a few more diets I have given a try for a short period of time. Low-carb diet, which comprised of low carbs overall, around 30–50g (per day), most of which were consumed early in the day, followed by high amounts of (lean) protein and moderate amounts of fat, with a total of five to six meals in a day. This was a hard diet to follow, and although it accelerated weight loss, it was tough to maintain.

Keto (ketogenic) diet, which comprised of very low carbs overall, around 30g (per day), mainly from low glycemic index foods, followed by high amounts of (healthy) fats and moderate amounts of protein, with a total of four to five meals a day or having meals when hungry. It was the hardest diet I tried. Although it resulted in accelerated weight loss (comparatively), it was also quite tough to maintain.

Carb-cycling diet, alternating days with low and high amounts of carbs. For example, days one to three were comprised of relatively low carbs, around 100–150g, followed by a day or two of higher carbs, around 200–300g, while keeping protein and fat intake moderate. I would continue a cycle of low and high carb days. It was an interesting diet, however, was slightly challenging to keep track of variations. It did not work out so well for me, and was not easy to maintain.

BRIEF SUMMARY:

- There are so many types of diets, it comes down to which one is suitable, works best, and is maintainable (after trying it).

TWO SS–SUGAR AND SALT

What I have learned is there are two culprits, added sugar and salt (sodium), which when consumed in relatively high quantity can interfere with weight loss and possibly lead to weight gain. Added sugar refers to sugar which has been added to a food product and is not naturally occurring within the food. Consider added sugar amongst the top main culprits, since it's contained in a lot of foods we typically consume. It does not really have much nutritional benefits or values. Cane sugar or corn syrup (substituted for sugar) is created through a process, meaning they do not occur naturally in that form. When sugary foods are consumed, they can give a rapid surge of energy (short term) followed by a sluggish feeling later, not to mention the possible health related risks associated with excess consumption of added sugar (and its equivalents) getting stored as fat. Therefore, knowing this, removing salt and added sugar should be the easiest thing to significantly reduce within a diet. Reducing these two then results in reduction of the overall excess caloric intake.

Be mindful of food items that contain added sugar. For example, a single-serving of ketchup (one tablespoon) may contain roughly four grams of sugar, which is about one teaspoon of sugar. Let's say three tablespoons of ketchup are consumed, that would mean about one tablespoon of sugar. That's a significant amount of sugar. There are other perhaps not so obvious foods which may contain plenty of sugar, such as drinks, flavored syrups, premade or bottled coffee and tea, chocolate spreads, cereal, BBQ sauce, flavored milk/milkshakes.

A method I use to help be mindful about added sugar is to do a quick conversion of sugar, typically listed in grams on nutritional labels, into teaspoons or tablespoons of sugar (one teaspoon ≈ four grams; one tablespoon ≈ twelve grams). For example, if eating a food item containing 24g of sugar per serving, first convert the quantity to nearest teaspoons and/or tablespoons. In this case, it equates to around six teaspoons, or two tablespoons of sugar. Now visualize the quantity, then imagine eating that much sugar by itself. How would it feel? Most likely not so great. Now, consider all of that added sugar is in whichever food item is being thought about being eaten. Think of processed sugar with a different perspective—it does not seem to be all that necessary, otherwise it would have existed naturally.

To spot added sugar on nutritional labels, look for sugar, cane sugar, corn syrup, high fructose corn syrup, cane juice, or similar additives. There are some countries that do not use high fructose corn syrup, and some corn can be genetically modified (GMO = Genetically Modified Organism). Do a little research prior to consuming foods containing high fructose corn syrup and genetically modified ingredients.

Regular sodas typically contain a lot of added sugar. Just read the nutrition label to see how many grams (g) of sugar there are, and do a similar conversion to the one mentioned earlier, this one into teaspoons or tablespoons. Popular sodas with a serving size of twelve fluid ounces (355 mL) can contain up to 40g or more of sugar! This would mean approximately ten teaspoons, or more than three tablespoons of sugar. Imagine eating this much sugar by itself. How would it feel? Most likely not so good. Now realize all that sugar is within the soda.

After learning this information, I decided to slowly reduce my consumption of soda, which eventually led me to exclude it from my diet all together. Sugar-eating thought process: If you cannot or would not want to eat the overall equivalent sugar by itself, then why eat it in a combined form with the food? Is it necessary? How about taking one or two small bites of an added sugar-containing food item and allow a couple minutes to settle in, then the craving might be minimized.

As I was reducing my intake of regular soda, I would sometimes substitute it with diet soda. Consequently, I started to consume diet soda. However, after being aware and learning artificial sweeteners commonly found in diet sodas (such as aspartame) are not such a healthy alternative, I followed a similar gradual approach as I did regular soda and eventually excluded diet soda from my diet as well.

Soda or drink alternatives: What I choose over sodas and other drinks with added sugar. For instance, when eating out or at a restaurant, I go for sparkling or soda water and sometimes add lemon and/or lime as a substitute for soda. Or just get plain water and add lemon and/or lime. For drinks, I typically select pure 100% fruit juices and try to avoid drinks made from concentrate or which have added sugar. Other options include coconut water and fruit and/ or vegetable smoothies without added sugar, in moderate quantities.

Salt, also commonly known as table salt (sodium chloride), is added to food typically for flavor, seasoning, or as a preservative, though some foods naturally contain sodium. Although sodium is a necessity, it can occur in high quantities in certain types of common foods. High sodium in a diet is considered unhealthy and may potentially lead to health risks. In contrast, your body also needs potassium, which might often be ignored or not known about. A variety of foods contain potassium, such as vegetables, fruits, and whole foods.

If, for instance, the suggested daily sodium intake limit is about 2,300 milligrams (mg) or 2.3 grams (g), this would be around one teaspoon (approximately 5.7 grams) of table salt. It's good to remember this as a reference. It's easy to see how much sodium there is in a food by reading the *Nutritional Label* and looking for sodium along with the percentage associated with it to know how much sodium there is per serving size.

Most of the salt appears to come from processed or packaged foods. Here are a few examples: fast foods, processed meat (such as hot dogs, smoked meat, deli meat, etc.), canned food (such as soup and vegetables), frozen meals, certain snacks, processed cheese, sauces (such as soy sauce) and certain dressings, and seasonings are some examples of foods that can contain high amounts of salt/sodium.

Aside from learning there might be potential health risks associated with high intake of sodium, I noticed reducing it aided with weight loss as well. Therefore, I got cautious of foods which contained high amounts of sodium.

Table salt is typically processed. Natural alternatives include Himalayan pink salt, Celtic salt, or sea salt. When cooking meals at home, I tend to use these types of salt instead.

✦ **Tip:** When going to restaurants look at nutritional information beforehand and check to see how much sodium and sugar there is for any dish that might be selected. Note, this information is usually available on the internet by searching for the restaurant name followed by "nutritional information." Unlike food nutritional labels, this nutrition information may not have percentages listed, therefore it may be helpful to remember sodium and sugar related amounts and correlations mentioned earlier for making a sound decision.

BRIEF SUMMARY:

- Be mindful when selecting drinks and foods, as some may contain lots of sugar and sodium.
- Check the *Nutrition Label* and *Ingredients List* for sugar and sodium.
- Some alternatives for table (or processed) sugar are honey, maple syrup, date sugar, and coconut sugar in moderation or small quantitics.
- Some alternatives for table salt (sodium) are Himalayan pink salt, Celtic salt, or sea salt (in moderation).
  - Spices, herbs, and seasonings can be used for food flavoring.

EATING OUT AND GROCERY SHOPPING

It was initially challenging not knowing what to order when eating out at a restaurant or with family or friends. What I've learned over time is to plan ahead whenever possible. Before going, I would look up the menu and nutritional information to decide on a couple options. Those options were mainly salads. An interesting general observation: When looking at the nutritional information for salads, usually the overall calories, including dressing, would be similar to some other dishes/meals on the menu. Typically, a good chunk of the calories within a salad would come from the dressing. Hence, when ordering a salad I would request the dressing on the side and used very little of it. Or sometimes requested for a different, lower calorie, dressing on the side.

If salad was not an option, I would select grilled or baked options. For example, a grilled fish and sides like grilled or steamed vegetables, bakes potato over mashed potatoes, steamed rice over fried rice, etc. As far as dessert was concerned, it would just be skipped. Sometimes I might take just one or two small bites from a shared dessert. For drink, like the alternatives mentioned in the previous chapter, I would get water with lemon or lime. If fresh fruit juice was an option I occasionally select it instead.

When having food at friend's or family's place, depending on the food options available, I took an informed and a healthier approach, keeping portion size in check while avoiding fried or greasy options and dessert. For instance, choosing vegetables over other side options and fruit over dessert if available. For ideas, refer to the "Carbs, Protein, and Fat" section in the "Diet" chapter.

Grocery shopping can get tricky, especially when there are so many options available.

✦ **Tip:** Avoid going grocery shopping when hungry. I have noticed shopping for groceries while hungry may lead to the purchase of unnecessary and/or excessive items. When navigating through the grocery, I would avoid processed foods/meats and pre-packaged meals. As an example, refer to the food items listed in the "Diet" chapter under "Carbs, Protein and Fat" section along with the "Supplementary Food and Snacks" list. Read the nutritional label in a similar way as described in Chapter Two, "Nutrition Essentials." Try to pick non-GMO and/ or organic food options as much possible.

Brief Summary:

- Plan ahead when eating out, look up menu and nutritional information in advance for restaurants. Make mindful meal choices while keeping portion sizes in check.
- Avoid grocery shopping on an empty stomach or when hungry.
- Avoid processed food/meat.
- Choose whole and organic food options.
- Read the *Nutrition Label* and *Ingredients List* before selecting a food product.

Food Awareness and Healthy Living

In today's world, with so many food options it's important to understand and have proper awareness of the food being consumed. Here is a list of items to be considerate and mindful about:

- Pre-packaged processed foods: These typically contain several ingredients, which can be found on the *Ingredients List*, including preservatives. May also contain high amounts of sugar, sodium, and fat.

- Foods containing unnatural preservatives: Preservatives should be listed in the *Ingredients List*. Think about the meaning of the word "preserve" and it's purpose. Now, how would that affect the digestion, breakdown, and absorption of food when it's trying to preserve food?

- Non-organic chicken and eggs: It may no longer be a great source for protein. After researching how chickens are treated I excluded non-organic chicken and eggs from my diet.

- Processed meats (such as lunch/deli meats, hot dogs): Processed meats may contain harmful chemicals and preservatives and be high in sodium.

- Foods high in sodium and sugar: Refer to the "Two Ss" chapter for more information.

- Artificial sweeteners: Commonly found in diet sodas and sugar-free food items.

- High fructose corn syrup: May add unnecessary unhealthy calories to the diet, which are converted to fat. Common foods which may contain high fructose corn syrup include soda, candy, yogurt.

- GMO (Genetically Modified Organism): Common examples can be corn, soy, and canola. Generally, these foods may not be labelled GMO.

   ○ There are certain countries where GMOs have been banned.

- Excessive meat: May bring large amounts of unhealthy fats. Also, check the *Nutrition Label* and notice the amount of cholesterol and its percentage per serving size. Check the *Nutritional Label*, for example, of chicken breast or fish, and there might be around 20% cholesterol per serving (depending on the weight).

- Hydrogenated oils: Created through a chemical process. If partially hydrogenated oil is listed on the ingredients list, then the food contains trans fat (which is not a healthy fat), despite the label reading 0 (zero) trans fat. This could be labelled this way as long as trans fat content is less than 0.5g per serving. Common examples include margarine, shortening, and baked food (pre-made type). Monoglycerides and diglycerides listed on the ingredients list may also contain trans fat.

- Microwave popcorn.

- Honey: Check ingredients. Some may contain added sweeteners, corn syrup, and/or sugar.

- Non-stick cookware.
- Low-fat or fat-free food: May contain sugar (or higher amount than healthier options), artificial sweeteners, additives.
- For further information, check with a healthcare or related professional.

HERE ARE USEFUL, HEALTHIER CHOICES AND TIPS:

- Instead of processed foods, try organic and non-GMO whole food, whole grains (100%), whole wheat, whole oats, brown rice, white rice, popcorn, beans, legumes, dairy products.
- Wild-caught seafood instead of farm raised, organic meats (lean/low fat) instead of non-organic.
  - ○ Although organic is generally more expensive, large quantities of meat are not so necessary.
- Instead of processed cane or corn sugar, try honey, maple syrup, date sugar, or coconut sugar (use in moderation, small quantities).
- Fiber has many benefits, naturally occurring in foods like fruits, vegetables, beans, legumes, and whole grains.

- Non-GMO, preferably organic, food options are healthiest.
- Wash fruits and vegetables before eating or soak them in water for few minutes. Vinegar or salt can be added to the water as well. Since not knowing exactly how they have been treated, it is best to wash fruits and vegetables before eating.
- Chew food serval times at a mild pace, helping with better digestion.
- Instead of frying food, save on excess calories by baking, grilling, or air frying.
- Drink water while sitting down, and at a mild pace.
- Natural cheese over processed cheese.
- Glass or stainless-steel food containers over plastic.
- Cast-iron, stainless steel and/or glass cookware over non-stick options.
- Keep stress as less as possible. Getting enough quality sleep, walking, or a warm bath may help reduce stress. Stress-relieving meditation or mindfulness is another avenue.
- Meat is not the only source for protein. Vegetables, legumes, beans, nuts, dairy food, whole grains, and many other non-meat food offer protein.

- Include cruciferous vegetables, such as cabbage, cauliflower, broccoli, Brussel sprouts, kale.
- Wash and dry hands with soap and water before eating. When water and soap are not available, hand sanitizer or hand rub (alcohol based) can be used.
- Shop at local farmers markets.

For more information, check with a healthcare or related professional.

Exercise/Workout

Exercise or workout categories I focused on were aerobic and anaerobic types of training. Aerobic exercise being with or in the presence of oxygen, using it to fuel energy. Common examples of cardiovascular exercises are brisk walking, running, biking, swimming. Anaerobic, being in the absence of oxygen, utilizing glucose for fuel. Common examples are weight/resistance training, sprinting, and high-intensity exercise for a short duration typically followed by a brief rest period.

My exercise routine was (aerobic) cardio in the morning on a fasted state to maximize fat burning, mainly using the treadmill, sometimes the elliptical machine. While exercising, the focus was to stay within a certain range of heartrate, approximately about 55 to 70 percent of the maximum heart rate, also commonly known as the fat-burning zone (utilizing fat for fuel). The idea was to burn a higher percentage of fat compared to other forms of exercise, like high intensity, which would most likely help burn more calories overall.

Fat-burning zone related information may also be listed on the treadmill, elliptical, or other machines. If not listed, here is a way to find out. First, know maximum heartrate (bpm—beats per minute), which is calculated by 220 minus your age. Multiply the result with 0.55 once, and then with 0.70. For example, max heart rate for a 35-year-old would be 220 minus 35, resulting in 185 bpm. Now, multiply 185 by 0.55, which gives 102 (rounded up), multiplied by 0.70, equaling 130 (rounded up), resulting in a heart range of 102–130 bpm. The goal would be to stay within this heartrate range while doing cardio.

To measure heartrate, a wristband-based fitness tracker, smart watch, or a similar device with a heartrate monitor may be used. To measure heartrate manually, lightly place middle and index finger on the inner side of the opposite wrist, under the thumb, or place both fingers on either side of the neck under the jawbone and feel the pulse. If the pulse is not felt, move the fingers slightly until felt. Now, with the help of a watch/clock, count the pulses for ten seconds. When finished counting, multiply the count by six, which will give you your heart rate. While on the treadmill, if my heart rate would be getting higher than expected (70 percent), I lowered the speed on the treadmill to stay within the desired heartrate range.

My cardio sessions typically lasted between ten and fifteen minutes, followed by weight/resistance workout. My workout plan will be mentioned on the upcoming pages, with the focus being on the major muscle groups. Between each set I would take a rest period of thirty seconds. On average, I would go to the gym about five days a week. In general, for workouts I learned it's not the amount of weight lifted that matters, it's actually the form and method that matters more (depending on the overall goal). The overall time I spent in the gym was around thirty to forty minutes. After about six or seven weeks of working out, I would take a week off from the gym to rest and recover.

Before starting a resistance/weights-related workout, I would start off with performing at least one or two warmup sets using a light weight. When performing an exercise with weights, for example doing a seated bicep curl using a dumbbell, I would slowly curl/lift the dumbbell up toward the shoulder while keeping the upper arm still and then slowly return to the starting position. The amount of weight I would use would be enough to allow ten repetitions easily, and then would slightly increase the weight for the second set and third set. I would avoid sudden or rapid movements and would remain focused on the muscle group that is being worked on. If I did not feel the intended muscle being under a little tension or strain, I would adjust the form, angle, or seat height as applicable.

When working out at a different time other than in the morning, I would at least maintain a gap of one to two hours or more after eating a meal before going to the gym. I learned that after working out, muscles need time to recover, taking up to two days for muscle recovery. Hence, I would not repeat the same type of workout on the following day. For example, if bicep curls were performed on day one, that same exercise or other exercise(s) utilizing the same muscle group would not be repeated on the following day.

On days I felt a little lazy and perhaps not in the mood for going to the gym, I would do listen to upbeat music or sometimes take a couple sips of coffee (without milk, creamer, and sugar) for a little energy. You can go outdoors instead, for example running or yoga outside. Also, utilizing the TV on the treadmill or elliptical machine for a little entertainment while working out can be helpful to keep you going.

Here are some ways I used to burn extra calories on random days: playing video games that involve physical motion (The types of games I played were sports and dance games, just to burn additional calories while having a little fun); at-home exercises based on videos; initially, when I did not have a gym membership, I started working out at the apartment gym. Sometimes I would go to outdoors for walking, jogging, running, and playing sports such as basketball to burn extra calories. Hiking was another option. I would take stairs instead of the elevator and parked further away to have a longer walk.

Occasionally, I would try high-intensity interval training (HIIT). It involves working out at a very high intensity for a short period of time. I would use the treadmill for it, starting with a brief warmup, then sprinting at a high speed for about thirty to sixty seconds or less, depending on how long I could withstand, followed by a minute of rest, which was walking on the treadmill at a low speed. I would then repeat this for a total of three to four times. It was a very intense form of exercise.

The appearance of muscle definition is generally related to body fat percentage. For instance, the abs (abdominal muscles) may not be visible due to a higher body fat percentage (fat covering the muscles). I have noticed as the body fat percentage is lowered as a result of losing weight (fat), muscle definition slowly begins to appear, giving a leaner and a more defined look. When seeing someone in person or on screen who is in a great shape, muscular and toned (muscles clearly visible), then most likely they would have a very low body fat percentage. What's interesting is if the same person gains weight, goes to a higher body fat percentage, their muscular definition (physique) would not appear the same way or as big as before, although their body size measurements would have increased, and may no longer appear very lean or muscular.

In short, it's the body fat percentage that changes the perception of physical appearance. When losing weight, I noticed fat from other areas of the body is reduced first, then the stomach/abdominal area. The opposite was true when a little weight was gained, in that it appeared to go around the stomach/abdominal area first instead of other areas.

Interesting fact, muscles can hold more weight in the eccentric phase of motion, which is when the muscle lengthens, which in a bicep curl exercise would be during the motion when the dumbbell is lowered downward.

When working out, muscle soreness may be experienced, especially during the first few times. When starting a workout plan, I would prefer to start with exercise machines as opposed to free weights, since they typically have a fixed range of motion and help concentrate on the intended muscle group(s). Then slowly with time, begin to incorporate free weights as desired. If any exercise is felt not comfortable or painful or shortness of breath is experienced, safely stop that exercise to avoid any risk of injury and seek help/assistance (as necessary). I would not overexert or over train when it came to exercise.

MY WORKOUT PLAN:

- **Arms (Biceps and Triceps) – 10 or 8 reps (repetitions)**
  - 2 warmup sets of either barbell or dumbbell curls (light weight)
  - 2 warmup sets for triceps, overhead dumbbell extension (light weight)
  - 3 sets of barbell curls
  - 3 sets of concentration curls
  - 3 sets of alternate dumbbell curls (seated)
  - 3 sets of standing triceps pushdown
  - 3 sets of lying forehead extension
  - 3 sets of standing overhead barbell extension

- **Chest – 10 or 8 reps**
  - 2 warmup sets on Pec Deck machine (light weight)
  - 3 sets of barbell bench press (flat bench)
  - 3 sets of incline barbell bench press
  - 3 sets of flat bench dumbbell fly
  - 3 sets of cable crossover (cable fly)

- **Back (Lats) – 10 or 8 reps**
  - ○ 2 warmup sets of lat pulldown (light weight)
  - ○ 3 sets of lat pulldown
  - ○ 3 sets of underhand cable pulldown
  - ○ 3 sets of seated cable rows
  - ○ 3 sets of dumbbell row

- **Shoulders – 10 or 8 reps**
  - ○ 2 warmup sets, alternative front shoulder raises and side dumbbell raises (light weight)
  - ○ 3 sets of seated dumbbell shoulder press
  - ○ 3 sets of barbell shoulder press
  - ○ 3 sets of side dumbbell raises
  - ○ 3 sets of alternating front dumbbell raises
  - ○ 3 sets of dumbbell rear delt fly

- **Legs – 10 or 8 reps**
  - ○ 2 warmup sets, squats (light weight)
  - ○ 3 sets of squats
  - ○ 3 sets of leg press
  - ○ 3 sets of leg extension
  - ○ 3 sets of leg curl
  - ○ 3 sets of seated calf raise

Now I only workout on average three days a week (alternate days), focusing mainly on resistance/weight training. The only cardio-type exercise I do is around ten to fifteen minutes of walking.

Brief Summary:

- There are several different methods and types of exercises and workouts.
  - ○ Gym, outdoor activities—hiking, sports, swimming—exercise videos, at-home workout, video games involving physical motion—dance, sports games—or simply walking.
- Personal training.
- Start with low intensity and low weights (preferably using exercise machines instead of free weights).
- Avoid repeating the same type of muscle group-related exercise on consecutive days.
- Get a good night sleep for rest and recovery.
- Avoid over training or overexertion.

FLEX DIET/SUSTAINABLE LIFESTYLE

By far this is my favorite kind of diet, which I use now if I would like to lose more weight or get leaner. It's a combination of intermittent fasting and three meals a day, beginning my morning with just a glass of water and staying in a fasted state (water would not break the fast due to 0 calories). I will have a late breakfast, somewhere between 8:30 and eleven in the morning (depending on how I am feeling and my hunger levels). The breakfast would be moderate in size, followed by a moderately heavy lunch a few hours later in the afternoon (or when hungry). My evening will start with a moderate to light dinner, preferably around six, or latest, seven. I will avoid snacking between breakfast, lunch, and dinner, though I may eat a small snack before going to the gym or working out, mainly for an energy boost (depending on how I would be feeling at that time). I always drink plenty of water throughout the day, even when not thirsty. I end with an intermittent fasting (non-eating) window of about 14–16 hours.

Diets should not necessarily have to be rushed in to when starting (unless needed). Hence, I prefer to ease into the diet, gradually reducing the number of overall meals in the day, with a similar approach for snacking in between meals, slowly increasing the intermittent fasting window. This window can also be a different window, or at a different time during the day.

Some benefits I noticed when comparing this type of diet to others, such as one which mentions consuming about six smaller sized meals throughout the day, is there is less meal preparation involved, and meals are more satisfying, as the portion size is not small. It's not restrictive on foods like carbs and requiring minimal or negligible amount of carb intake. You will not feel hungry all the time and will save time, as less time is spent toward cooking and eating. This plan is comparatively easier to manage, no calorie counting necessary. A flex diet is a more sustainable type of diet, and can therefore become a lifestyle.

MY DIET PLAN (EXAMPLE):

Meal 1 – Breakfast:
Typically one of the following three:

1. Two or three organic egg omelet (with vegetables) and two large or three small slices of whole grain bread.
2. About 1 & ½ cup whole grain cereal with minimal or no sugar added along with 1 cup of regular milk (organic).
3. 1 & ½ cup of steel-cut oatmeal (cooked) with ½ teaspoon of honey.

MEAL 2 – LUNCH:

Lunch is balanced combinations of carbs, protein, and fat options mentioned in the "Diet" chapter. Avoid processed, pre-packaged foods. I occasionally combine a snack mentioned in the "Snack" section of the "Diet" chapter with the lunch meal in small quantity. When having dessert cravings, I would eat fruit, half a cup or less of organic ice cream, or just half a teaspoon of honey, or one of the snack items. Combining snacks with a meal helped minimize any cravings later.

MEAL 3 – DINNER:

Dinner consists a lighter version of lunch, with the main focus on mixed vegetables seasoned and prepared several different ways, such as grilled, baked, or sometimes as a salad or soup.

SNACK – PRE-WORKOUT (TYPICALLY):

I may have a small snack, typically before going to the gym or workout. Refer to "Snack" section in the "Diet" chapter.

As part of this lifestyle, I do not have any cheat meals or days. Occasionally, when I would like to eat pizza, I would go with a thin crust, plain cheese, or with veggies, and keep portion size moderate. When craving a burger, I would go with a moderate-sized grilled (or charbroiled) option with a small quantity of sweet potato fries or substitute with a different side (with no soda or drinks). Similar concept when eating a pasta or lasagna, eating in moderation and choosing whole grain (or whole wheat) pasta. My preferred time for eating such a meal would be lunch, and key would be in moderation, which would help satisfy craving and food desires. As for desserts, I do not normally have a huge desire for, and when I do, I just grab a fruit or have a little dark chocolate instead. Otherwise, if I would really like to try an appealing dessert, I would just take no more than one or two small bites (this would not be very frequent).

Sometimes when I eat a larger than usual meal, then I go lighter on the next meal, or sometimes even skip it if I am not hungry. I have noticed meal or diet plans can be customized and changed if one does not work successfully or as needed.

After learning there are so many food sources other than meat containing protein, I no longer eat meat every single day (which also helps avoid the cholesterol that comes along with meat). On random days each week, I skip meat and choose plenty of other food options that contain protein.

Intermittent fasting is eating during a set window and fasting during the remaining window in a day (usually carrying over to the next day). Typically, a fasting window would be greater than twelve hours. I have noticed intermittent fasting has also helped me lose weight.

What is breakfast? Think about it as two words, "break" and "fast"—breaking the fast. Aren't we already fasting while sleeping or when we wake up? In the concept of intermittent fasting, one method is to just have a breakfast later in the morning or day, which would simply allow the fasting window to be extended after waking up. In usual routine, we are used to having a breakfast early morning, however, does is it really have to be early in the morning? Think about this from a slightly different perspective.

Brief Summary:

- Diet with three meals a day while avoiding snacking in between (combining snacks with meals if desired).
- Combining intermittent fasting (no eating window, except water—0 calories—with the diet as desired, perhaps having a late breakfast).
- Healthier eating. Choose whole foods and incorporate vegetables and fruit within the diet. Eat in moderation. Be creative with healthy food options for cooking and eating.

How to Get Started Today!

Consult with a physician (doctor) and preferably a dietitian.

1. Take body measurements: Waist _____ in, Chest _____ in, Hips _____ in, Thigh _____ in, Arms _____ in.
2. Starting weight: _____ (lb. or kg—circle one).
3. Take photos and save them.
4. Weight loss: Goal setting, short term: _____ (lb. or kg) and long term: _____ (lb. or kg).
5. a) Use a nutrition or calorie counter app (for example, MyFitnessPal) to track current food intake (calories). Otherwise, track calories manually by looking at food nutritional labels or by searching for food related caloric information on the app.

   Or

   b) Determine what the suggested maintenance calories to maintain current weight are. Typically, it's based on height, weight, gender, and other factors. Check whether the current (normal routine) daily overall caloric intake is higher or lower than the maintenance calories. If its higher, then the maintenance caloric value can be used as a starting point for daily caloric intake. If not higher, then just subtract about 400 calories from the maintenance calories, or as comfortable, and use that number as daily caloric threshold.

6. Choose any one of the diets mentioned while utilizing the overall information previously shared (as desired). Or try any other diet which may suit you better.

7. Slowly start to incorporate food changes using previously mentioned (healthier) food choices. Gradually clean out your pantry, fridge, and freezer from all the junk, processed foods.

8. Gently start decreasing consumption of food items with added sugar (or equivalent) and high sodium. In other words, gradually decrease added sugar and sodium intake.

9. Start tracking weight using either a calendar, an app, or the table provided on last pages for tracking weight. For weighing, I use a digital scale.

10. If starting an exercise or workout plan, consult/hire an experienced personal

trainer. If not an option, start with a friend or workout partner who has good experience.

- If no changes in weight are noticed in about a week, adjust overall caloric intake, most likely reducing calories, for example, by 100 calories or so. Review the food choices and adjust as needed.
- Remember to drink plenty of water throughout the day.

Although I only counted calories for a relatively short period of time, it was a very valuable learning experience. It brought a new perspective toward diet, and afterward helped me with being mindful with food choices and portion sizes.

Similarly, I hired a personal trainer for a short period of time (about two weeks) even though I had myself completed an entire personal training course. The personal trainer was highly experienced and had previously competed in bodybuilding championships. It was an immensely beneficial learning experience for me. Although personal training can be expensive, a lot can be learned. When thinking about personal training, it's imperative to hire an experienced personal trainer with whom you're comfortable with. Do a little research on personal training ahead of time and get referrals (if possible).

For weight measurement, timing is important and should be consistent. I chose early in the morning before eating/drinking anything for measuring weight, and remained consistent. Also, the amount of clothing worn can affect the weight on the scale.

When starting a new diet it takes a few days to get in to the routine, and the first couple of days may be slightly hard, but after that it doesn't feel that hard and becomes a routine. From my experience, weight loss is not a linear and predictable process. Remember the tips, ideas, and secrets shared within the book.

Start the diet gently and slowly, then slightly change it afterward when not seeing results. I wouldn't go at it full throttle or hard right away, ease into the new diet gently. With time your body adapts, so you may have to make little adjustments with your diet plan to avoid a plateau (if not noticing any change for a while). Slightly reduce overall caloric intake. Instead of being repetitive with the same types of food in a routine, keep changing it up, try to be creative. Similar with exercise and workouts, start mildly. Start with light weights when beginning an exercise routine, then over time gradually increase weights or intensity and duration along with frequency (depending on overall goal).

Breakdown overall weight loss goal in to smaller, short-term goals. For example, if overall goal is to lose twenty pounds, then a short-term goal can be ten pounds or smaller as desired. Once the short-term goal is reached, take body measurements and photo and compare with ones from before to note progress.

There are many healthy recipes with whole foods on the internet. It does take time in the kitchen to cook, however, think about how much time is spent doing other non-essential things like watching tv or spending time on the cell phone, looking up social media... How about diverting some of that non-essential time toward the kitchen (cooking) and healthier eating?

BRIEF SUMMARY:

- Refer to the step-by-step approach in this chapter.
- Weight loss (natural) is generally not a linear, overnight process, it's gradual.
- Keep track of weight, keeping timing consistent for when weighing.
  - Weigh at a minimum interval of a week or less if preferred (to keep close track).
- Slowly and gradually make changes in diet (as desired and/or needed).

- Counting calories is a valuable learning experience.
- Break down overall goal into smaller, short-term goals.
- Get a good night sleep (rest).
- If not exercising or working out, incorporate walking into your daily routine.

THE SECRET AND KEY INFORMATION

Here is my secret: dark chocolate. What I noticed is it helped me with suppressing the urge to overeat or overindulge, and also helped when desiring a dessert after a meal. For instance, after eating a preferred portion of lunch but still having a feeling to eat more, I would have a piece of 70% dark chocolate. Afterward, I would not have the feeling to eat more. Typically, I would not have dark chocolate with every single meal, just when desired.

When I tried less than 70% dark chocolate, it did not have the same effect. When trying higher than 70% dark chocolate, I noticed it did have the effect, but for me the taste was not very satisfying. Hence, I choose 70% (or close to 70%) dark chocolate. In general, I noticed dark chocolate has less sugar content when compared to regular milk chocolate.

Another key method which helped me with weight loss was drinking water shortly before a meal. Frequently, I would drink at least one, sometimes up to two glasses of water (approximate 8–16 ounces) to fill up a little before a meal. Occasionally, I would drink some water during a meal or as desired, but avoided drinking it right after finishing a meal. In between meal times, if I would start to feel a little hungry or craved a snack, I would drink one or two glasses of water and it would help suppress the sensation to snack or eat.

After eating a meal, give a few minutes to trigger hunger fullness instead of continuing to eat till perhaps the stomach is entirely full. After eating a meal, the feeling of fullness would not be instantaneous and would take a few minutes. So, sometimes after a meal I would just make myself busy to avoid the sensation to eat more, and consequently, after a few minutes the feeling of fullness would arrive and the desire to eat more would go away.

As previously mentioned, keeping only healthy snacking options around can help. Here is a different perspective on meals. We are used to eating at pre-set times like breakfast, lunch, and dinner, not eating when we are actually hungry. Think about preset eating times from a different perspective.

Calorie equality. Not all types of food calories are the same. For instance, 100 calories of candy will most likely not have the same effect and benefits as 100 calories worth of vegetables, which makes food choices significant.

Here is my breakdown for three major items pertaining to weight loss. For an understanding of how much significance each roughly has: Diet–70%, Sleep–15%, Exercise–15%.

Weight Loss (breakdown)

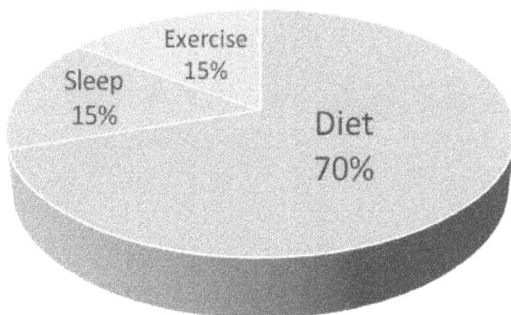

BRIEF SUMMARY:

- My secret: dark chocolate (70% or more). It helped me with suppressing the urge to overeat or overindulge or desire a post-meal dessert.
- Drinking water shortly before a meal and plenty throughout the day.
- Get a good night sleep (rest).
- Calorie equality. Not all types of food calories are the same. For instance, 100 calories of candy will most likely not

have the same effect and benefits as 100 calories of vegetables.

- My breakdown for three major items pertaining to weight loss: Diet–70%, Sleep–15%, and Exercise–15%.

Motivation

L ooking for motivation for losing weight? Here are a few examples: to be healthier, be in a better shape, would like clothes to fit better, would like to do it for yourself, for someone special or family, improve confidence, or other. List one or more here_____ _____.

After losing weight, it simply felt amazing. It made me passionate about diet, health, and fitness. I noticed my confidence was boosted and I felt much happier and had more energy throughout the day. Clothes also fit so much better.

One day when I was carrying a five-gallon water bottle up the stairs, the noticeable weight of the bottle (approximately 42 pounds) made me think as a reference that before losing weight I was carrying around more than twice the equivalent amount of extra weight. I then wondered how that much extra weight affected the joints and the body overall internally. Imagine how good the feeling might be when that extra weight is lost.

The thought is not to let food cravings be in control. Instead, you need to be in control of food. Remain disciplined with your diet and be patient. Weight loss is sort of dynamic, not linear, and with time may get slower as body fat is reduced. Remain consistent and patient and results will come.

Seeing results over time and seeing the number reduce on the scale should be a great motivator to keep going and continue losing fat. Getting good comments or complements from people should motivate even further. Finding a role model, maybe someone who has lost weight can be an inspiration too. There were a few people who inspired me with their dedication and exemplary levels of fitness.

To get motivated for working out, or to get yourself going, you can listen to a song you like or an updated playlist. Or look at a picture of a fitness person you like or follow on social media and use that to motivate yourself to go to the gym.

Sometimes food temptations may be hard to resist. Choose ready-to-eat healthy snacks and keep the portion size very small depending on the type of food.

Let's think about it from a different perspective. No matter what the current situation is, take a moment to imagine, *What if it would have been worse?* For instance, if someone is currently twenty pounds overweight, what if it was forty pounds instead? But it isn't. So, do not feel terrible about it, leave that aside and get started. The time is now to make a change and be healthier.

It may take some months, or perhaps a year or more, to achieve your weight loss goal. This may sound like a lot, but within a lifetime span it's just a fraction. So, spending time doing a little effort now should not be much when compared to a lifespan. How about just doing it once in your lifetime, then sustain it and simply enjoy.

Be happy and content with however much weight loss has been achieved over time, even if the goal has not been met. If you feel like taking a break after a while, take a little break and go to a maintenance diet where you can increase calories and have a little recharge, and then get back on the diet while maintaining your current weight.

Flex diet (mentioned in the previous chapter) is not just a diet but a sustainable lifestyle for me by adjusting meal portion sizes to either maintain or lose weight further.

Do not be discouraged or disappointed with your weight. Stay happy, and more important, be patient, and never give up or lose hope.

Wishing you happiness and success.

TABLES FOR TRACKING WEIGHT

Sunday	Monday	Tuesday	Wednesday	Thursday	Friday	Saturday
Date:	Date:	Date:	Date:	Date:	Date:	Date:
Weight:	Weight:	Weight:	Weight:	Weight:	Weight:	Weight:
Date:	Date:	Date:	Date:	Date:	Date:	Date:
Weight:	Weight:	Weight:	Weight:	Weight:	Weight:	Weight:
Date:	Date:	Date:	Date:	Date:	Date:	Date:
Weight:	Weight:	Weight:	Weight:	Weight:	Weight:	Weight:
Date:	Date:	Date:	Date:	Date:	Date:	Date:
Weight:	Weight:	Weight:	Weight:	Weight:	Weight:	Weight:
Date:	Date:	Date:	Date:	Date:	Date:	Date:
Weight:	Weight:	Weight:	Weight:	Weight:	Weight:	Weight:
Date:	Date:	Date:	Date:	Date:	Date:	Date:
Weight:	Weight:	Weight:	Weight:	Weight:	Weight:	Weight:

Sunday	Monday	Tuesday	Wednesday	Thursday	Friday	Saturday
Date:	Date:	Date:	Date:	Date:	Date:	Date:
Weight:	Weight:	Weight:	Weight:	Weight:	Weight:	Weight:
Date:	Date:	Date:	Date:	Date:	Date:	Date:
Weight:	Weight:	Weight:	Weight:	Weight:	Weight:	Weight:
Date:	Date:	Date:	Date:	Date:	Date:	Date:
Weight:	Weight:	Weight:	Weight:	Weight:	Weight:	Weight:
Date:	Date:	Date:	Date:	Date:	Date:	Date:
Weight:	Weight:	Weight:	Weight:	Weight:	Weight:	Weight:
Date:	Date:	Date:	Date:	Date:	Date:	Date:
Weight:	Weight:	Weight:	Weight:	Weight:	Weight:	Weight:
Date:	Date:	Date:	Date:	Date:	Date:	Date:
Weight:	Weight:	Weight:	Weight:	Weight:	Weight:	Weight:

Sunday	Monday	Tuesday	Wednesday	Thursday	Friday	Saturday
Date:	Date:	Date:	Date:	Date:	Date:	Date:
Weight:	Weight:	Weight:	Weight:	Weight:	Weight:	Weight:
Date:	Date:	Date:	Date:	Date:	Date:	Date:
Weight:	Weight:	Weight:	Weight:	Weight:	Weight:	Weight:
Date:	Date:	Date:	Date:	Date:	Date:	Date:
Weight:	Weight:	Weight:	Weight:	Weight:	Weight:	Weight:
Date:	Date:	Date:	Date:	Date:	Date:	Date:
Weight:	Weight:	Weight:	Weight:	Weight:	Weight:	Weight:
Date:	Date:	Date:	Date:	Date:	Date:	Date:
Weight:	Weight:	Weight:	Weight:	Weight:	Weight:	Weight:
Date:	Date:	Date:	Date:	Date:	Date:	Date:
Weight:	Weight:	Weight:	Weight:	Weight:	Weight:	Weight:

Sunday	Monday	Tuesday	Wednesday	Thursday	Friday	Saturday
Date:	Date:	Date:	Date:	Date:	Date:	Date:
Weight:	Weight:	Weight:	Weight:	Weight:	Weight:	Weight:
Date:	Date:	Date:	Date:	Date:	Date:	Date:
Weight:	Weight:	Weight:	Weight:	Weight:	Weight:	Weight:
Date:	Date:	Date:	Date:	Date:	Date:	Date:
Weight:	Weight:	Weight:	Weight:	Weight:	Weight:	Weight:
Date:	Date:	Date:	Date:	Date:	Date:	Date:
Weight:	Weight:	Weight:	Weight:	Weight:	Weight:	Weight:
Date:	Date:	Date:	Date:	Date:	Date:	Date:
Weight:	Weight:	Weight:	Weight:	Weight:	Weight:	Weight:
Date:	Date:	Date:	Date:	Date:	Date:	Date:
Weight:	Weight:	Weight:	Weight:	Weight:	Weight:	Weight:

Sunday	Monday	Tuesday	Wednesday	Thursday	Friday	Saturday
Date:	Date:	Date:	Date:	Date:	Date:	Date:
Weight:	Weight:	Weight:	Weight:	Weight:	Weight:	Weight:
Date:	Date:	Date:	Date:	Date:	Date:	Date:
Weight:	Weight:	Weight:	Weight:	Weight:	Weight:	Weight:
Date:	Date:	Date:	Date:	Date:	Date:	Date:
Weight:	Weight:	Weight:	Weight:	Weight:	Weight:	Weight:
Date:	Date:	Date:	Date:	Date:	Date:	Date:
Weight:	Weight:	Weight:	Weight:	Weight:	Weight:	Weight:
Date:	Date:	Date:	Date:	Date:	Date:	Date:
Weight:	Weight:	Weight:	Weight:	Weight:	Weight:	Weight:
Date:	Date:	Date:	Date:	Date:	Date:	Date:
Weight:	Weight:	Weight:	Weight:	Weight:	Weight:	Weight:

Sunday	Monday	Tuesday	Wednesday	Thursday	Friday	Saturday
Date:	Date:	Date:	Date:	Date:	Date:	Date:
Weight:	Weight:	Weight:	Weight:	Weight:	Weight:	Weight:
Date:	Date:	Date:	Date:	Date:	Date:	Date:
Weight:	Weight:	Weight:	Weight:	Weight:	Weight:	Weight:
Date:	Date:	Date:	Date:	Date:	Date:	Date:
Weight:	Weight:	Weight:	Weight:	Weight:	Weight:	Weight:
Date:	Date:	Date:	Date:	Date:	Date:	Date:
Weight:	Weight:	Weight:	Weight:	Weight:	Weight:	Weight:
Date:	Date:	Date:	Date:	Date:	Date:	Date:
Weight:	Weight:	Weight:	Weight:	Weight:	Weight:	Weight:
Date:	Date:	Date:	Date:	Date:	Date:	Date:
Weight:	Weight:	Weight:	Weight:	Weight:	Weight:	Weight:

Sunday	Monday	Tuesday	Wednesday	Thursday	Friday	Saturday
Date:	Date:	Date:	Date:	Date:	Date:	Date:
Weight:	Weight:	Weight:	Weight:	Weight:	Weight:	Weight:
Date:	Date:	Date:	Date:	Date:	Date:	Date:
Weight:	Weight:	Weight:	Weight:	Weight:	Weight:	Weight:
Date:	Date:	Date:	Date:	Date:	Date:	Date:
Weight:	Weight:	Weight:	Weight:	Weight:	Weight:	Weight:
Date:	Date:	Date:	Date:	Date:	Date:	Date:
Weight:	Weight:	Weight:	Weight:	Weight:	Weight:	Weight:
Date:	Date:	Date:	Date:	Date:	Date:	Date:
Weight:	Weight:	Weight:	Weight:	Weight:	Weight:	Weight:
Date:	Date:	Date:	Date:	Date:	Date:	Date:
Weight:	Weight:	Weight:	Weight:	Weight:	Weight:	Weight:

70

Sunday	Monday	Tuesday	Wednesday	Thursday	Friday	Saturday
Date:	Date:	Date:	Date:	Date:	Date:	Date:
Weight:	Weight:	Weight:	Weight:	Weight:	Weight:	Weight:
Date:	Date:	Date:	Date:	Date:	Date:	Date:
Weight:	Weight:	Weight:	Weight:	Weight:	Weight:	Weight:
Date:	Date:	Date:	Date:	Date:	Date:	Date:
Weight:	Weight:	Weight:	Weight:	Weight:	Weight:	Weight:
Date:	Date:	Date:	Date:	Date:	Date:	Date:
Weight:	Weight:	Weight:	Weight:	Weight:	Weight:	Weight:
Date:	Date:	Date:	Date:	Date:	Date:	Date:
Weight:	Weight:	Weight:	Weight:	Weight:	Weight:	Weight:
Date:	Date:	Date:	Date:	Date:	Date:	Date:
Weight:	Weight:	Weight:	Weight:	Weight:	Weight:	Weight:

Sunday	Monday	Tuesday	Wednesday	Thursday	Friday	Saturday
Date:	Date:	Date:	Date:	Date:	Date:	Date:
Weight:	Weight:	Weight:	Weight:	Weight:	Weight:	Weight:
Date:	Date:	Date:	Date:	Date:	Date:	Date:
Weight:	Weight:	Weight:	Weight:	Weight:	Weight:	Weight:
Date:	Date:	Date:	Date:	Date:	Date:	Date:
Weight:	Weight:	Weight:	Weight:	Weight:	Weight:	Weight:
Date:	Date:	Date:	Date:	Date:	Date:	Date:
Weight:	Weight:	Weight:	Weight:	Weight:	Weight:	Weight:
Date:	Date:	Date:	Date:	Date:	Date:	Date:
Weight:	Weight:	Weight:	Weight:	Weight:	Weight:	Weight:
Date:	Date:	Date:	Date:	Date:	Date:	Date:
Weight:	Weight:	Weight:	Weight:	Weight:	Weight:	Weight:

Sunday	Monday	Tuesday	Wednesday	Thursday	Friday	Saturday
Date:	Date:	Date:	Date:	Date:	Date:	Date:
Weight:	Weight:	Weight:	Weight:	Weight:	Weight:	Weight:
Date:	Date:	Date:	Date:	Date:	Date:	Date:
Weight:	Weight:	Weight:	Weight:	Weight:	Weight:	Weight:
Date:	Date:	Date:	Date:	Date:	Date:	Date:
Weight:	Weight:	Weight:	Weight:	Weight:	Weight:	Weight:
Date:	Date:	Date:	Date:	Date:	Date:	Date:
Weight:	Weight:	Weight:	Weight:	Weight:	Weight:	Weight:
Date:	Date:	Date:	Date:	Date:	Date:	Date:
Weight:	Weight:	Weight:	Weight:	Weight:	Weight:	Weight:
Date:	Date:	Date:	Date:	Date:	Date:	Date:
Weight:	Weight:	Weight:	Weight:	Weight:	Weight:	Weight:

Sunday	Monday	Tuesday	Wednesday	Thursday	Friday	Saturday
Date:	Date:	Date:	Date:	Date:	Date:	Date:
Weight:	Weight:	Weight:	Weight:	Weight:	Weight:	Weight:
Date:	Date:	Date:	Date:	Date:	Date:	Date:
Weight:	Weight:	Weight:	Weight:	Weight:	Weight:	Weight:
Date:	Date:	Date:	Date:	Date:	Date:	Date:
Weight:	Weight:	Weight:	Weight:	Weight:	Weight:	Weight:
Date:	Date:	Date:	Date:	Date:	Date:	Date:
Weight:	Weight:	Weight:	Weight:	Weight:	Weight:	Weight:
Date:	Date:	Date:	Date:	Date:	Date:	Date:
Weight:	Weight:	Weight:	Weight:	Weight:	Weight:	Weight:
Date:	Date:	Date:	Date:	Date:	Date:	Date:
Weight:	Weight:	Weight:	Weight:	Weight:	Weight:	Weight:

Sunday	Monday	Tuesday	Wednesday	Thursday	Friday	Saturday
Date:	Date:	Date:	Date:	Date:	Date:	Date:
Weight:	Weight:	Weight:	Weight:	Weight:	Weight:	Weight:
Date:	Date:	Date:	Date:	Date:	Date:	Date:
Weight:	Weight:	Weight:	Weight:	Weight:	Weight:	Weight:
Date:	Date:	Date:	Date:	Date:	Date:	Date:
Weight:	Weight:	Weight:	Weight:	Weight:	Weight:	Weight:
Date:	Date:	Date:	Date:	Date:	Date:	Date:
Weight:	Weight:	Weight:	Weight:	Weight:	Weight:	Weight:
Date:	Date:	Date:	Date:	Date:	Date:	Date:
Weight:	Weight:	Weight:	Weight:	Weight:	Weight:	Weight:
Date:	Date:	Date:	Date:	Date:	Date:	Date:
Weight:	Weight:	Weight:	Weight:	Weight:	Weight:	Weight:

Sunday	Monday	Tuesday	Wednesday	Thursday	Friday	Saturday
Date:	Date:	Date:	Date:	Date:	Date:	Date:
Weight:	Weight:	Weight:	Weight:	Weight:	Weight:	Weight:
Date:	Date:	Date:	Date:	Date:	Date:	Date:
Weight:	Weight:	Weight:	Weight:	Weight:	Weight:	Weight:
Date:	Date:	Date:	Date:	Date:	Date:	Date:
Weight:	Weight:	Weight:	Weight:	Weight:	Weight:	Weight:
Date:	Date:	Date:	Date:	Date:	Date:	Date:
Weight:	Weight:	Weight:	Weight:	Weight:	Weight:	Weight:
Date:	Date:	Date:	Date:	Date:	Date:	Date:
Weight:	Weight:	Weight:	Weight:	Weight:	Weight:	Weight:
Date:	Date:	Date:	Date:	Date:	Date:	Date:
Weight:	Weight:	Weight:	Weight:	Weight:	Weight:	Weight:

73

Sunday	Monday	Tuesday	Wednesday	Thursday	Friday	Saturday
Date:	Date:	Date:	Date:	Date:	Date:	Date:
Weight:	Weight:	Weight:	Weight:	Weight:	Weight:	Weight:
Date:	Date:	Date:	Date:	Date:	Date:	Date:
Weight:	Weight:	Weight:	Weight:	Weight:	Weight:	Weight:
Date:	Date:	Date:	Date:	Date:	Date:	Date:
Weight:	Weight:	Weight:	Weight:	Weight:	Weight:	Weight:
Date:	Date:	Date:	Date:	Date:	Date:	Date:
Weight:	Weight:	Weight:	Weight:	Weight:	Weight:	Weight:
Date:	Date:	Date:	Date:	Date:	Date:	Date:
Weight:	Weight:	Weight:	Weight:	Weight:	Weight:	Weight:
Date:	Date:	Date:	Date:	Date:	Date:	Date:
Weight:	Weight:	Weight:	Weight:	Weight:	Weight:	Weight:

Sunday	Monday	Tuesday	Wednesday	Thursday	Friday	Saturday
Date:	Date:	Date:	Date:	Date:	Date:	Date:
Weight:	Weight:	Weight:	Weight:	Weight:	Weight:	Weight:
Date:	Date:	Date:	Date:	Date:	Date:	Date:
Weight:	Weight:	Weight:	Weight:	Weight:	Weight:	Weight:
Date:	Date:	Date:	Date:	Date:	Date:	Date:
Weight:	Weight:	Weight:	Weight:	Weight:	Weight:	Weight:
Date:	Date:	Date:	Date:	Date:	Date:	Date:
Weight:	Weight:	Weight:	Weight:	Weight:	Weight:	Weight:
Date:	Date:	Date:	Date:	Date:	Date:	Date:
Weight:	Weight:	Weight:	Weight:	Weight:	Weight:	Weight:
Date:	Date:	Date:	Date:	Date:	Date:	Date:
Weight:	Weight:	Weight:	Weight:	Weight:	Weight:	Weight:

74

www.ingramcontent.com/pod-product-compliance
Lightning Source LLC
Chambersburg PA
CBHW022127280326
41933CB00007B/575